The Whole Body Reset:

I0479244

Your Weight reduction Technique for Flat Belly and a Healthy Feeling

By

James C. Stanley

Introduction:

Quite possibly the most well-known objective that individuals set for themselves is to shed pounds. As a rule, as people, we generally make progress toward a sound and fit way of life. Large numbers of us, nonetheless, come up short on inspiration and expertise to seek after such objectives. Moreover, not every person has the strength or discipline to see things through once they begin. It ought not to be challenging to see the reason why this is the situation regards to decreasing weight and staying fit. No question about taking that part in unsafe ways of behaving like gorging or basic lying more pleasant. However, numerous people are ignorant that the method involved with being fit and solid may likewise be pleasant. In all actuality, that is the way to long haul outcome in excess fit and solid. Everything revolves around making the method as euphoric and energizing as could be expected, so you stay enchanted all through.

CHAPTER 1

12 TIPS TO HELP YOU lOSE WEIGHT

1. Try not to skip breakfast

Skipping breakfast won to assist you with getting thinner. You could pass up fundamental supplements and you might wind up eating no question taking since you feel hungry.

2. Eat normal feasts

Eating at normal times during the day helps consume calories at a quicker rate. It likewise diminishes the impulse to nibble on food sources high in fat and sugar.

3. Eat a lot of products of the soil

Leafy foods are low in calories and fat, and high in fiber - 3 fundamental elements for fruitful weight reduction. They additionally contain a lot of nutrients and minerals.

4. Get more dynamic

Being dynamic is vital to getting in shape and keeping it off. As well as giving loads of medical advantages, exercise can assist with consuming the abundance of aloof rise you can't lose through diet alone.

Find an action you appreciate and can squeeze into your daily schedule.

5. Drink a lot of water

Individuals once in a while mistake hunger for hunger. You can wind up polishing off additional calories when a glass of water is truly what you want.

6. Eat high-fiber food sources

Food sources containing loads of fiber can assist with keeping you feeling full, which is ideal for getting thinner. Fiber is just tracked down in food from plants, like products of the soil, oats, wholegrain bread, earthy-colored rice and pasta, and beans, peas, and lentils.

7. Peruse food marks

Knowing how to peruse food names can assist you with picking better choices. Utilize the calorie data to resolve how a specific food squeezes into your everyday calorie recompense on the weight reduction plan.

8. Utilize a more modest plate

Utilizing more modest plates can assist you with eating more modest segments. By using more modest plates and bowls, you might have the option to bit by bit become accustomed to eating more modest parts without going hungry. It requires around 20 minutes for the stomach to tell the cerebrum it's fully complete eat gradually and quit eating before you feel full.

9. Try not to boycott food sources

Restrict no food varieties from your weight-reduction plan, particularly the ones you like. Prohibiting food sources will just cause them to desire them. There's no great explanation you can't partake in a periodic treat as long as you stay inside your day day-day-to-calorieompense.

10. Try not to stock unhealthy food

To keep away from allurement, don't stock low-quality food - like chocolate, rolls, crisps, and sweet bubbly es - at home. All things considered, choose solid tidbits, for example, natural products, unsalted rice cakes, oat cakes, unsalted or unsweetened popcorn, and organic product juice.

11. Eliminate liquor

A standard glass of wine can contain however many calories as a piece of chocolate. Over the long run, drinking an excess of the can without much of a stretch add to weight gain.

12. Plan your feasts

Attempt to design your morning meal, lunch, supper, and snacks for the week, ensuring you adhere to your calorie remittance. You might find it supportive to make a week-by-week shopping list.

CHAPTER 2

10 Encouraging Signs of Progress on Your Weight Loss Journey

10 signs you're losing weight

How might you tell that your well-being is consistently improving and your weight reduction venture is advancing? Here are a few eleearthy-coloredstrate that you're moving in a decent course:

1. You're not eager constantly

Assuming you're getting in shape since you changed your eating routine to incorporate more proteins and fewer carbs and fat, you might see that you feel full more quickly.

That is because the amino acids in dietary protein convey a fulfillment message to your mind — and that sign isn't sent by eating a similar number of calories in fat or carbs.

The uplifting news here for veggie lovers and vegetarians: A recent report found that the fulfillment signal is more grounded with vegetable proteins and creature-inferred inferred proteins.

2. Your feeling of prosperity gets to the next level

Getting in shape can prompt an overall improvement in your mental well-being. In a recent report Believed Source, individuals who were attempting to get thinner detailed that they felt greater essentialness, more restraint, less sadness, and less uneasiness than they had felt before their weight reduction.

On the off chance that you're not feeling these profound advantages yet, don't surrender: Study members didn't report this enhancement half-year point The enormous mental changes appeared at the year interviews. Another significant that if you're getting in shape as an unexpected symptom of injury, sickness, or a major life-altering separation-employment cutback, you probably won't encounter a similar profound upsurge.

3. Your garments fit in an unexpected way

You might see that you don't need to leap to pull on your pants, even before you see a major distinction on the scale — which can inspire you to continue doing what you're doing. In 2017, around 77% of ladies and 36 percent of men said they were persuaded to get fitter to develop further how their garments fit their bodies.

4. You're seeing some muscle definition

It can require some investment — generally weeks or months — to develop fortitude and see muscle definition. How quickly you see changes will rely upon your body and the sort of activity you've integrated into your arrangement. In 2019 concentrate by Believed Source found that young ladies fabricated more bulk in their legs when they performed more redundancies of leg twists and presses with a lighter burden than with lefewereps and a heavier burden.

To continue to construct muscle as you shed pounds, specialists suggest Confided in Source that you get enough (yet not to an extreme) protein and do obstruction type works out.

5. Your body estimations are evolving

A contracting midriff size uplifting news for your general well-being. Researchers followed 430 individuals in a 2-year weight the executive's program and noticed that a decrease in midsection estimation was related to our developed results in pulse, glucose, and cholesterol. Other studies have drawn an immediate connection between your midriff outline and your gamble of cardiovascular infection. Whether the scale expresses you're down, a looser belt implies better heart well-being. Your persistent aggravation moves along

Weight reduction can assist with diminishing torment, particularly in the weight-bear regions of the body, similar to the lower legs and lower back. In one 2017 review, individuals who lost something like 10% of their body weight saw the best improvement in ongoing torment around weight-bearing zones. One losing 20% of body weight emphatically further developed knee torment and irritation in individuals with joint pain.

7. You're going to the restroom more — or less — much of the time

Changing what you eat may influence your defecation designs.

Disposing of meat and adding more mixed greens and vegetables to your eating routine can further develop clogging. However, adding more creature protein to your eating routine (as numerous paleo and keto consume fewer calories do) can make certain individuals more inclined to blockage. If you're worried about the distinctions in your defecations, or on the other hand on the off chance that they're slowing down your efficiency, it could be smart to consult with a nutritionist or medical care supplier about tweaking your arrangement to further develop your stomach wellbeing.

8. Your circulatory strain is descending

Being overweight can hurt your circulatory strain, making you defenseless against strokes and coronary episodes. One method for cutting down your circulatory strain is to shed pounds with a better eating regimen and greater development. Assuming that you're getting fitter, you're lessening the burden on your heart and starting to standardize your pulse.

9. You wheeze less

Wheezing has a convoluted relationship with weight. Scientists have tracked down that individuals (particularly ladies) who have metabolic conditions (a forerunner to diabetes) will generally wheeze. Wheezing and rest apnea might try and cause weight gain. Hence, weight reduction is many times one of the designated treatments for individuals who wheeze and who have dozing messes.

10. Your state of mind moves along

Rolling out sound improvements to your dietary patterns can prompt a superior state of mind and more energy. In 2016, specialists found that a high glycemic load diet comprising of treats, potatoes, wafers, cakes, and bagels, which will generally cause spikes in glucose, prompted 38% more side effects of sadness and 26 percent more exhaustion than a low glycemic load diet. Assuming your food decisions are causing fewer pinnacles and valleys in your glucose, you're presumably feeling a portion of the profound and mental advantages that come from weight reduction.

What are a few signs that you're getting in shape excessively quickly?

Seeing a major weight change in a brief period might be exceptionally persuasive, however shedding pounds through a trend to eat fewer carbs or unreasonable practices can cause a few unfortunate secondary effects, for example,

- fatigue

- slowed metabolism

- muscle cramps

- gallstones

- weakened immune system

If you're not sure about the long-term health effects of your weight management plan, talk with a registered dietitian, a licensed nutritionist, or your healthcare provider about it early in your process.

CHAPTER 3

Top 12 Biggest Myths About Weight Loss

1. All calories are equivalent

The calorie is an estimation of energy. All calories have a similar energy content. Nonetheless, this doesn't imply that all calorie sources affect your weight. Various food varieties go through various metabolic pathways and can affect hunger and the chemicals that direct your body weight.

For instance, a protein calorie isn't equivalent to a fat or carb calorie.

Supplanting carbs and fat with protein can support your digestion and decrease hunger and desires, all while improving the capability of some weight-controlling chemicals.

Additionally, calories from entire food varieties like organic products will generally be substantially more filling than calories from refined food varieties, like treats.

2. Getting thinner is a straight cycle

As certain individuals suspect, getting fitter is normally not a straight interaction.

Occasionally and weeks you might get in shape, while during others you might acquire a tad.

This isn't a reason to worry. It's typical for body weight to change all over by a couple of pounds.

For instance, you might be conveying more food in your stomach-related framework or clutching more water than expected.

This is considerably more articulated in ladies, as water weight can vary fundamentally during the feminine cycle (4Trusted Source).

However long the general pattern is going downwards, regardless of the amount it vacillates, you will in any case prevail with regards to getting in shape over the long haul.

3. Enhancements can assist you with getting in shape

The weight reduction supplement industry is gigantic. Different organizations guarantee that their enhancements make emotional impacts, yet they're seldom extremely powerful when considered. The primary explanation that enhancements work for certain individuals is a self-influenced consequence. Individuals succumb to the advertising strategies and believe that the enhancements should assist them with getting thinner, so they become more aware of what they eat.

All things considered, a couple of enhancements unassumingly affect weight reduction. The best ones might assist you with shedding a modest quantity of weight for more than a while.

4. Heftiness is about determination, not science

It is erroneous to say that your weight is about determination.

Corpulence is an exceptional mind mind-boggling with handfuls — on the off chance that not hundreds — of contributing elements.

Various hereditary factors are related to heftiness, and different ailments, like hypothyroidism, PCOS, and melancholy, can expand your gamble of weight gain. Your body likewise has various chemicals and natural pathways that should direct body weight. These will more often than not be useless in individuals with heftiness, making it a lot harder to get in shape and keep it off.

For instance, being impervious to the chemical leptin is a significant reason for stoutness. The leptin signal should let your mind know that it has sufficient fat put away. However, assuming you're impervious to leptin, your cerebrum feels that you're starving. Attempting to apply self-control and deliberately eating less notwithstanding the leptin-driven starvation signal is unimaginably troublesome. This doesn't imply that individuals ought to surrender and acknowledge their hereditary destiny. Getting in shape is as yet conceivable — it's only a lot harder for certain individuals.

Outline

Corpulence is a mind-boggling problem. Numerous hereditary, organic, and ecological variables influence body weight. Thusly, shedding pounds isn't just about resolution.

5. Eat less, move more

The muscle-to-fat ratio is just putting away energy. To lose only, want to consume a bigger number of calories than you take in. Hence, it appears to be just legitimate that eating less and moving more would cause weight reduction.

While this guidance works in principle, particularly if you make an extremely durable way of life change, it's a terrible proposal for those with a serious weight issue. A great many demands this guidance wind up recovering any shed pounds because of physiological and biochemical elements. A significant and supported real context conduct is expected to get fitter with diet and exercise. Confining your food admission and enticement to get more actual work. Teaching somebody with stoutness to just eat less and move more resembles advising somebody with despondency to encourage or body liquor addiction to drink less.

Synopsis

Advising individuals with weight issues to simply eat less and move more is incapable of guidance that seldom works in the long haul.

6. Carbs make you fat

Low-carb diets can help with weight reduction.

By and large, this happens even without cognizant calorie limitation. However long you keep carb admission low and protein consumption high, you'll get in shape. All things being equal, this doesn't imply that carbs cause weight gain. While the stoutness pestilence began around 1980, people have been eating carbs for quite a while.

Entire food varieties that are high in carbs are exceptionally solid.

Then again, refined carbs like refined grains and sugar are connected to weight gain.

Outline

Low-carb consumes fewer calories and is exceptionally viable for weight reduction. Be that as it may, carbs are not what causes heftiness in any case. Entire, single-fixing carb-based food varieties are extraordinarily solid.

7. Fat makes you fat

Fat gives around 9 calories for each gram, contrasted and just 4 calories for every gram of carbs or protein. Fat is very calorie-thick and typical in low-quality foods. However, as long as your calorie admission is inside a sound reach, fat doesn't make you fat.

Furthermore, eating fewer carbs that are high in fat yet low in carbs has been displayed to cause weight reduction in various examinations. While loading your eating routine with unfortunate, unhealthy low quality foods weighed down with fat will make you fat, this macronutrient isn't the sole offender.

Your body needs sound fats to appropriately work.

Synopsis: Fat has frequently been faulted for the stoutness plague. While it adds to your absolute calorie consumption, fat alone doesn't cause weight gain.

8. Having breakfast is important to shed pounds

Concentrates on a show that morning meal captains will generally weigh more than breakfast eaters. Be that as it may, this is presumable because individuals who have breakfast are bound to have another propensity. In the A month concentrate 309 grown-ups thought about breakfast propensities and found no impact on weight or whether the members had or skipped breakfast. Likewise, a legendary breakfast helps digestion and various little dinners cause you to consume more calories over the course of the day. It's ideal to eat when you're ravenous and stop when you're full. Have breakfast when you need to, yet don't anticipate that it should significantly affect your weight.

Synopsis

While it is the case that morning meal captains will generally weigh more than breakfast eaters, controlled investigations show that whether you have or skip breakfast doesn't make any difference in weight reduction.

9. Cheap food is continuously stuffing

Not all cheap food is undesirable.

Given individuals' expanded well-being cognizance, many cheap food chains have begun offering better choices. Some, for example, Chipotle, even spotlight solely on serving quality food sources.

It's feasible to get something somewhat solid at most cafés. Most modest drive-thru eateries frequently give better options in contrast to their principal contributions.

These food varieties may not fulfill the requests of every wellbeing cognizant individual, yet they're as yet a respectable decision if have the opportunity or energy to prepare a quality dinner.

Rundown

Cheap food doesn't need to be undesirable or swell. Most inexpensive food chains offer a few better options in contrast to their principal contributions.

10. Weight reduction consumes fewer calories work

The weight reduction industry believes that you should accept that diets work. Notwithstanding concentrating on showing that consuming fewer calories seldom works in the long haul. Prominently, 85% of calorie counters wind up recovering load soon. Also, studies demonstrate that individuals who diet are probably going to put on weight from now on. Consequently, consume less calories are a steady indicator of future weight gain — not misfortune. Truly you likely shouldn't move toward weight reduction with a slimming down mentality. All things considered, make it an objective to change your way of life for all time and become a better, more joyful, and fitter individual. If you figure out how to build your activity levels, activity, and rest better, you ought to get in shape as a characteristic secondary effect. Consuming fewer calories likely won't work in the long haul.

11. Individuals with corpulence are unfortunate and dainty individuals are solid

Heftiness without a doubt expands your gamble of a few constant sicknesses, including type 2 diabetes, coronary illness, and a few diseases.

Be that as it may, a lot of individuals with heftiness are metabolically sound and a lot of slim individuals have these equivalent ongoing infections.

It appears to issue where your fat develops. If you have a ton of fat in your stomach region, you're at a more serious gamble of metabolic sickness.

Synopsis

Stoutness is connected to a few persistent illnesses, like sort 2 diabetes. In any case, many individuals with weight are metabolically sound, while many slim individuals are not.

12. Diet food sources can assist you with getting fit

A great deal of low-quality food is showcased as sound. Models incorporate low-fat, sans-fat, and handled without-gluten food sources, as well as high-sugar drinks. You ought to have some serious doubts about well-being claims on food bundling, particularly on handled things. These names for the most part exist to hoodwink — not inform. Some unhealthy food advertisers will urge you to purchase their swelling low-quality food If the bundling of goods lets you know that it's sound, there's an opportunity it's the specific inverse.

CHAPTER 4

20 Best Superfoods for Weight reduction

"Superfoods" is a word frequently utilized for supplement-rich fixings that give significant medical advantages. Other than advancing in general well-being, numerous superfoods contain explicit mixtures, cancer prevention agents, and micronutrients that might upgrade weight reduction.

The following are 20 of the best superfoods for weight reduction, all supported by science.

1. Kale

Kale is a verdant green vegetable that is notable for its wellbeing advancing properties.

It's an incredible wellspring of cancer prevention agents and a few key supplements, including manganese and nutrients C and vitamin K . Kale is likewise low in calories and high in fiber, a compound that moves gradually through the gastrointestinal system and helps keep you feeling more full for longer, which might uphold weight reduction.Have a go at adding kale to your #1 serving of mixed greens, sautéing it with garlic for a simple side dish, or utilizing it to add a pop of variety to pasta dishes.

2. Berries

Berries like strawberries, blueberries, and blackberries are dynamic, tasty, and exceptionally nutritious. For instance, blueberries are plentiful in fiber and nutrients C and K. They can likewise assist with fulfilling your sweet tooth while giving fewer calories than numerous other high-sugar tidbits or pastries. Berries function admirably in smoothies or as fixings for yogurt or cereal. They likewise make a fantastic tidbit, either all alone or joined with different natural products in an organic product salad.

3. Broccoli

Broccoli is a supplement thick superfood and a great expansion to a sound weight reduction diet. Specifically, broccoli is an extraordinary wellspring of fiber and micronutrients, like L-ascorbic acid, folate, potassium, and manganese. Various investigations additionally show that increasing your admission of cruciferous vegetables, including broccoli, could assist with forestalling weight gain over the long haul. Add a touch of garlic, lemon juice, or Parmesan — or each of the three — to your broccoli for a speedy and simple side dish. You can likewise have a go at adding broccoli to plates of mixed greens, meals, quiches, or pasta dishes to increase their health benefit.

4. Chia seeds

Chia seeds are stacked with significant supplements, including omega-3 unsaturated fats, calcium, magnesium, and manganese. They're likewise loaded with dissolvable fiber, which is a sort of fiber that retains water and structures a gel in the gastrointestinal system. Research recommends that consuming solvent fiber might be connected to expanded weight reduction and muscle-to-fat ratio misfortune. Chia seeds are additionally high in protein, which can assist with lessening hunger and managing your craving. Have a go at sprinkling chia seeds over your #1 smoothies, yogurts, or oat bowls to upgrade the flavor and surface.

5. Eggs

Eggs are flexible, flavorful, and easy to get ready. It's not difficult to see the reason why they're one of the most outstanding superfoods for weight reduction.

Eggs are loaded with various fundamental nutrients and minerals in each serving, including selenium, vitamin B12, riboflavin, and phosphorus. Moreover, eggs are overflowing with protein, which can assist with elevating sensations of completion to help weight reduction.

Hard-bubbled eggs make an incredible tidbit sprinkled with some salt and pepper or a touch of hot sauce. You can likewise appreciate eggs in omelets, quiches, breakfast burritos, and pan-sears.

6. Avocado

Avocados are famous for their extraordinary taste and surface, as well as their amazing supplement profile. Specifically, avocados are high in potassium, folate, and nutrients C and K.

Even though avocados are viewed as a calorie-thick food, they're stacked with fiber and heart-solid unsaturated fats, which can keep you feeling full between dinners to assist you with getting thinner. Avocados can bring a velvety surface and rich flavor to toast, mixed greens, soups, or fried eggs. They additionally make an amazing option for sauces and fortunes like guacamole, hummus, and salsa.

7. Yams

Yams are an energetic, tasty, and nutritious superfood.

They're stacked with cancer prevention agents, alongside nutrients An and C, manganese, and B nutrients. Also, yams are high in fiber, which can ease back stomach discharging to support both weight reduction and fat misfortune. You can heat, squash, bubble, or sauté yams and appreciate them as a filling tidbit or side dish.

8. Kimchi and sauerkraut

Kimchi is a typical fix in Korean food. It regularly comprises ted, aged vegetables like cabbage and radish.

Sauerkraut is the European adaptation of this dish, likewise regularly made with matured cabbage.

Like other matured food varieties, kimchi and sauerkraut are extraordinary wellsprings of probiotics. These are a sort of useful microorganisms likewise tracked down in your stomach, and they support a few parts of well-being.

Curiously, a few examinations recommend that probiotic enhancements might assume a part in weight guidelines and influence hunger and sensations of totality. To fit more probiotics into your eating routine, take a stab at eating kimchi with rice or adding it to stews, grain bowls, or noodle dishes. Sauerkraut works out in a good way in wraps and burgers and close-by frankfurters, including vegetarian assortments. It likewise coordinates well with cheddar.

There are no principles for how to eat kimchi and sauerkraut, so go ahead and explore different avenues regarding your food pairings. Many individuals additionally eat them all alone.

While you're picking kimchi and sauerkraut, keep away from assortments that contain added additives or sugar, as well as those that have been sanitized. Thoroughly search in the refrigerated segment of your supermarket.

You can likewise effectively make your kimchi or sauerkraut at home.

9. Chime peppers

Likewise in some cases alluded to as sweet peppers, ringer peppers are profoundly nutritious veggies accessible in different varieties.

They're wealthy in fiber and gloat a variety of other significant supplements, including L-ascorbic acid, vitamin B6, and potassium

.

On account of their high water content, they're likewise extremely low in calories and can supplant different fixings in your eating routine to diminish your day-to-day calorie admission and backing weight reduction. Match chime peppers with hummus, tzatziki, or yogurt plunge for a fast and simple low-calorie nibble. On the other hand, have a go at dicing them and adding them to soups, mixed greens, or pan-sears to light up your dishes.

10. Chickpeas

Chickpeas, otherwise called garbanzo beans, are a kind of vegetable firmly connected with different sorts of beans, including kidney beans, dark beans, and pinto beans.

Each serving of chickpeas is high in manganese, folate, phosphorus, and copper.

Chickpeas are additionally high in fiber and protein, which can slow processing, control your hunger, and advance weight reduction.

You can trade chickpeas in for different wellsprings of protein in feasts to give any recipe a plant-based contort. You can likewise heat or meal chickpeas and season them with your number one flavors for a basic bite.

11. Apples

Apples are not just perhaps of the most famous natural product on earth yet additionally one of the most nutritious. Apples are stuffed with cell reinforcements, in addition to fundamental micronutrients like L-ascorbic acid and potassium. They likewise contain a particular kind of solvent fiber called gelatin, which creature studies have shown may assist with diminishing food admission and increment weight reduction. Studies have proposed that remembering apples for a solid eating regimen might advance weight reduction and work on your general well-being. You can appreciate apples in their entire, crude structure for a sound, high-fiber nibble. They're likewise scrumptiously cut up and matched with peanut butter, cream cheddar, or yogurt plunge.

12. Spinach

Spinach is a famous verdant green vegetable initially from old Persia. It's low in calories and high in fiber, nutrients C and A, and iron. Likewise, spinach contains thylakoids, which are a kind of plant compound that might postpone fat processing and decrease yearning and desires. Notwithstanding mixed greens, there are a lot of other imaginative ways of adding spinach to your eating routine. Take a stab at adding it to pan-sears, soups, smoothies, or pasta dishes to carry some additional variety and micronutrients to your feast.

13. Pecans

The Image Storage room/Offset Pictures

Pecans are a sort of tree nut known for containing numerous sound supplements.

Alongside being wealthy in omega-3 unsaturated fats, pecans contain a concentrated measure of vitamin E, folate, and copper.

Even though they're somewhat high in calories, concentrates show w that the body retains 21fewerss calories from pecans than anticipated in light of their dietary benefit.

Studies have likewise shown that pecans might decrease cravings and hunger, which could be useful for long-haul weight reduction.

Pecans are perfect for adding a heart-sound mash to plates of mixed greens, grains, cereal, or yogurt. You can likewise prepare and toast them for a scrumptious, filling nibble.

14. Oats

Oats are an entire grain food and a cherished breakfast staple. Their logical name is Avena sativa.

They're a decent wellspring of fiber, manganese, phosphorus, copper, and protein.

On account of the ample protein and fiber in oats, they might be helpful for weight executive and craving control, as per a few examinations.

Other than oats, you can likewise appreciate oats in yogurt, smoothies, porridge, or heated merchandise.

15. Tomatoes

Tomatoes are a tart, tasty superfood and a fantastic expansion to a balanced weight reduction diet.

Tomatoes are likewise jam-loaded with cell reinforcements and nutrients and minerals, including nutrients C and K and potassium.

Furthermore, as a result of their high water content, tomatoes have a low-calorie thickness, which could assist with supporting long-haul weight reduction.

Tomatoes can add a hurdle of flavor to plates of mixed greens, wraps, and sandwiches. You can likewise utilize them to prepare tasty soups, sauces, salsas, and jams.

16. Green tea

Green tea is an intense wellspring of infection battling polyphenols and cell reinforcements.

Specifically, green tea is wealthy in cell reinforcements like quercetin, chlorogenic corrosive, and theogallin.

It's additionally high in epigallocatechin gallate (EGCG), a cell reinforcement that may he

CHAPTER 5

What medications are approved for weight loss?

Several drugs have been approved by the Food and Drug Administration (FDA) for weight loss for those over weigh obesity. These medications require a prescription from a doctor and should only be taken under medical supervision.

These include:

orlistat (Xenical)

phentermine/topiramate (Qsymia)

naltrexone/bupropion (Contrave)

glucagon-like peptide 1 (GLP-1) agonists, including liraglutide (Saxenda) and liraglutide (Wegovy)

setmelanotide (Imcivree)

appetite suppressants, including phentermine (Adipex-P or Lomaira), benzphetamine (Regimex or Didrex), diethylpropion (Tepanil or Tenuate), and phendimetrazine (Bontril)

These medications should be combined with a balanced weight loss diet, as they are not likely a helpful long-term solution to obesity and may lead to weight regain over time. They also have many possible side effects, some of which can be serious.

Prescription weight loss drugs

A quick look at prescription weight loss medications

- orlistat

- phentermine/topiramate

- naltrexone/bupropion

- GLP-1 agonists

- bremelanotide

- appetite suppressants

1. Orlistat (Xenical)

Orlistat is an oral medication that is available via prescription as Xenical. It can also be purchased over the counter as the brand Alli.

After a medical consultation, a doctor can prescribe orlistat. Certain telehealth services can also provide a prescription for this medication.

How it works: Orlistat works by blocking the activity of certain enzymes used to break down fats in the digestive tract, which helps to reduce the number of calories that you absorb.

Effectiveness: According to a 2011 study of 80 people with obesity, those who took orlistat lost an average of 10.3 pounds (lb), or 4.65 kilograms (kg), after 6 months. They also experienced significant reductions in body mass index (BMI), belly fat, and total and LDL (bad) cholesterol levels.

Side effects: Orlistat often causes digestive issues like loose or oily stools, gas, and frequent bowel movements. It could also contribute to nutrient deficiencies, including in fat-soluble vitamins A, D, E, or K. Following a low-fat diet is typically recommended while taking this medication to help minimize adverse side effects.

2. Phentermine/topiramate (Qysmia)

Phentermine/topiramate is an oral medication that belongs to a class of drugs known as sympathomimetic amines. It requires a prescription from a doctor and is sold under the brand, Qysmia.

How it works: This medication includes phentermine, a central nervous system stimulant and appetite suppressant with similar mechanisms to amphetamine. It also includes topiramate, an anticonvulsant that helps reduce appetite and enhance satiety to promote weight loss.

Effectiveness: One review concluded that phentermine/topiramate resulted in an average weight loss of 17 lb (7.7 kg) and significantly reduced belly fat, blood pressure, blood sugar, and cholesterol levels

Another review comparing the effectiveness of several weight loss medications found that people with overweight or obesity who took phentermine/topiramate lost an average of 19.4 lb (8.8 kg) after 1 year.

Side effects: The most common side effects associated with phentermine/topiramate include dry mouth, constipation, paresthesia, or a sensation of pins and needles.

It could also cause increased body temperature, an inability to sweat, and psychiatric or cognitive disturbances.

3. Naltrexone/bupropion (Contrave)

This medication, sold under the name Contrave, is an oral medication that combines bupropion, an antidepressant, and naltrexone, which is used to manage opioid or alcohol use disorder.

A doctor can determine whether Contrave may be a good option for you and may provide a prescription. Some online services may also prescribe Contrave following a virtual consultation with a healthcare professional.

How it works: Though the exact mechanism of naltrexone/bupropion is not fully understood, it's believed to promote weight loss by acting on certain parts of the brain to reduce food intake, boost metabolism, and increase feelings of fullness.

Effectiveness: One review of four studies showed that naltrexone/bupropion was associated with significant weight loss compared to a placebo. Over 1 year, participants lost an average of 11–22 lb (5–9 kg).

Another review had similar findings, reporting that naltrexone/bupropion could be effective for long-term weight loss maintenance as well.

Side effects: Naltrexone/bupropion may cause nausea, constipation, headache, vomiting, dizziness, and insomnia. It might also increase heart rate and blood pressure.

4. GLP-1 agonists

dzika_mrowka/Getty Images

Two GLP-1 agonists have been approved for weight loss, including liraglutide (Saxenda) and liraglutide (Wegovy). Both are available as a self-administered injection, but liraglutide is administered once daily while semaglutide is only injected once per week.

Though not approved specifically for weight loss, some other GLP-1 agonists intended to treat type 2 diabetes are also sometimes prescribed off-label for weight management, including:

- semaglutide (Ozempic or Rybelsus)
- dulaglutide (Trulicity)

- liraglutide (Victoza)

- exenatide (Byetta)

- exenatide extended-release (Bydureon BCise)

- tirzepatide (Mounjaro)

GLP-1 agonists are only available through a prescription from a doctor. Several telehealth services and weight loss programs can also provide a prescription if you meet the eligibility criteria, including Ro Body Program and Calibrate.

How it works: GLP-1 agonists work by slowing the emptying of the stomach, increasing feelings of fullness, and reducing the secretion of glucagon, a hormone involved in regulating appetite.

Effectiveness: Several studies have found that GLP-1 agonists could be beneficial for weight management.

For instance, one study in 1,961 adults found that taking 2.4 milligrams (mg) of semaglutide per week combined with lifestyle changes resulted in a nearly 15% reduction in body weight after 68 weeks.

Another small study found that people taking liraglutide lost an average of 17.2 lb (7.8 kg) over 6 months.

Side effects: Common side effects include nausea, vomiting, diarrhea, dizziness, headaches, increased heart rate, infections, and indigestion.

Though uncommon, severe side effects have also been reported, which may require medical attention, including kidney problems, thyroid C-cell tumors, gallbladder disease, low blood sugar, and suicidal ideation.

More research is also needed on the long-term effects of these medications, as there is concern about potential weight regain over time.

5. Setmelanotide (Imcivree)

Setmelanotide, sold as Imcivree, is in a class of medications known as melanocortin 4 (MC4) receptor agonists. It's an injectable medication approved for treating obesity caused by certain genetic mutations and is available only via prescription.

How it works: People with specific genetic mutations may experience insufficient activation of the MC4 receptor in the brain, which could contribute to obesity.

Setmelanotide works by increasing the activation of this receptor, leading to reduced hunger, decreased calorie intake, and increased metabolism, all of which could promote weight loss.

Effectiveness: One study in 21 people taking bremelanotide found that around 62% of participants achieved at least 10% weight loss after 1 year. Participants also experienced a significant reduction in hunger with no serious treatment-related adverse events reported.

Another small study in children, adolescents, and adults found that bremelanotide significantly improved quality of life as early as 5 weeks after starting treatment, which could be related to reduced hunger and body weight.

Side effects: Some of the most common side effects of setmelanotide include injection site reactions, hyperpigmentation, nausea, headache, diarrhea, and stomach or back pain. Fatigue, vomiting, and depression have also been reported.

6. Appetite suppressants

There are several anorectics, or appetite suppressants, available, including phentermine (Adipex-P or Lomaira), benzphetamine (Regimex or Didrex), diethylpropion (Tepanil or Tenuate), and phendimetrazine (Bontril).

These are all taken orally and require a prescription from a doctor or other healthcare professional.

How it works: These medications reduce appetite by altering levels of certain neurotransmitters in the brain, which can lead to weight loss.

Effectiveness: One study in 3,411 people compared the effectiveness of several medications for obesity and found that people taking phentermine lost the highest percentage of body weight over 12 weeks. Those taking phentermine lost an average of 8.3 lb (3.75 kg) throughout the study.

Another 2015 study in 156 people with obesity showed that people taking diethylpropion lost an average of 10.8 lb (4.9 kg) after 3 months and 17 lb (7.7 kg) after 6 months.

However, keep in mind that these medications are only recommended for short-term use, as you can build up a tolerance after several weeks, resulting in decreased effectiveness.

Side effects: Potential side effects of these medications may include nausea, vomiting, diarrhea, and stomach cramps.

Other severe side effects have also been reported and require immediate medical attention, including shortness of breath, chest pain, and swelling of the lower extremities.

Over-the-counter weight loss pills and supplements

A quick look at OTC weight loss pills

- garcinia cambogia extract
- Hydroxycut
- green coffee bean extract

- caffeine

- orlistat (Alli)

- raspberry ketones

- glucomannan

- meratrim

- green tea extract

- conjugated linoleic acid

- forskolin

- bitter orange/synephrine

1. Garcinia cambogia extract

Garcinia cambogia became popular worldwide after being featured on "The Dr. Oz Show" in 2012.

It's a small, green fruit shaped like a pumpkin. The fruit's skin contains hydroxy citric acid, the active ingredient in garcinia cambogia extract, which is marketed as a diet pill.

How it works: Animal studies show that it can hinder a fat-producing enzyme in the body and increase serotonin levels, potentially helping to reduce cravings.

Effectiveness: According to one meta-analysis of 54 studies, researchers found that garcinia cambogia had no significant effect on body weight or body fat percentage compared to a placebo.

On the other hand, a 2020 review that looked at eight trials on garcinia cambogia found that, on average, it caused weight loss of about 3 lb (1.34 kg).

Side effects: While it's widely agreed that garcinia cambogia is safe to take in recommended amounts, studies within the last several years have pointed to some serious side effects.

A 2018 study documented four cases of women who experienced acute liver failure after taking weight loss supplements containing garcinia cambogia.

Additionally, hepatotoxicity, liver impairment, and some episodes of mania have also been reported in conjunction with taking garcinia cambogia.

2. Hydroxycut

Hydroxycut has been around for more than a decade and is one of the most popular weight loss supplements in the world. The brand makes several products, but Hydroxycut is the most common.

How it works: It contains several ingredients claiming to help with weight loss, including caffeine and a few plant extracts such as green coffee extract.

Effectiveness: A 2011 meta-analysis of five clinical trials found that supplementation with C. canephora robusta, or green coffee extract, one of the key ingredients in Hydroxycut, led to about a 5.5-lb (2.47-kg) weight loss compared to the placebo.

Side effects: If you are sensitive to caffeine, you may experience anxiety, jitteriness, tremors, headaches, dizziness, and dehydration.

Hydroxycut products containing ephedra, a stimulant herb, were removed from shelves due to cardiovascular risks in 2004 and hepatotoxicity in 2009.

Acute liver injury has also been linked to using Hydroxycut supplements).

3. Green coffee bean extract

Green coffee beans are coffee beans that haven't been roasted. They contain two substances believed to help with weight loss, including caffeine and chlorogenic acid.

How it works: Caffeine can increase fat burning, and chlorogenic acid can slow the breakdown of carbohydrates in the gut.

Effectiveness: Several human studies have shown that green coffee bean extract could help people lose weight.

A meta-analysis of all the current randomized control trials on green coffee bean extract's effect on obesity found that the supplement has a significant impact on minimizing body mass index.

Other benefits: Green coffee bean extract may help lower blood sugar levels and reduce blood pressure. It is also high in antioxidants.

Side effects: It can cause the same side effects as caffeine. The chlorogenic acid it contains may also cause diarrhea, and some people may be allergic to green coffee beans.

4. Caffeine

Caffeine is the most commonly consumed psychoactive substance in the world. It is found naturally in coffee, green tea, and dark chocolate and is added to many processed foods and beverages.

Because caffeine is considered a metabolism booster, companies commonly add it to commercial weight loss supplements.

How it works: One study discussed the effect of caffeine on regulating body weight by increasing energy expenditure — essentially meaning you burn more calories via increased fat breakdown and through a process of body heat production called thermogenesis.

Effectiveness: Some studies show that caffeine can cause modest weight loss in humans.

Side effects: In some people, high amounts of caffeine can cause anxiety, insomnia, jitteriness, irritability, nausea, diarrhea, and other symptoms. Caffeine is also addictive and can reduce the quality of your sleep.

There is no need to take a supplement or a pill containing caffeine. The best sources are quality coffee and green tea, which have antioxidants and other health benefits.

5. Orlistat (Alli)

Orlistat is a pharmaceutical drug sold over the counter under the brand name Alli and via prescription as Xenical.

How it works: This weight loss pill works by inhibiting the breakdown of fat in your gut, meaning that you take in fewer calories from fat.

Effectiveness: A 2003 meta-analysis of studies found that people taking orlistat for 12 months in combination with lifestyle changes saw a 2.9% greater weight reduction than the placebo group. However, there are no recent studies to confirm the drug's effectiveness.

Other benefits: Orlistat has been shown to reduce blood pressure slightly and may reduce the risk of developing type 2 diabetes when used alongside lifestyle changes.

Side effects: This drug has many digestive side effects, including loose, oily stools, flatulence, and frequent bowel movements that are hard to control. It may also contribute to a deficiency in fat-soluble vitamins such as vitamins A, D, E, and K (4).

Following a low-fat diet while taking orlistat is often recommended to minimize side effects. Interestingly, a low-carb diet (without medication) has been considered as effective as an orlistat and a low-fat diet combined.

Both diets were as effective for weight loss but showed no significant differences in blood sugar and blood lipid levels. However, orlistat combined with a low-carb diet was more effective at lowering blood pressure.

6. Raspberry Ketones

Raspberry ketone is a substance found in raspberries and is responsible for their distinct smell.

A synthetic version of raspberry ketones is sold as a weight loss supplement.

How it works: In isolated fat cells from mice, raspberry ketones increase the breakdown of fat and increase levels of a hormone called adiponectin, which is believed to be related to weight loss.

Effectiveness: Though there are very few studies on raspberry ketones in humans, one 2013 study looked at raspberry ketones with some other ingredients and found a potential 2% increase in weight loss over 8 weeks when compared with a placebo.

Another mouse study using massive doses showed some delay in weight gain. However, high doses of raspberry ketones were also associated with higher blood sugar levels and higher levels of ALT, a liver enzyme, indicating liver dysfunction.

It's unknown whether these effects would translate to humans. More research is necessary to determine any benefits and risks.

Side effects: According to some anecdotal reports, raspberry ketones can cause your burps to smell like raspberries.

In animal studies, high doses were also associated with increased blood sugar levels and liver dysfunction, though more research in humans is needed.

7. Glucomannan

Glucomannan is a type of fiber found in the roots of the elephant yam, which is also called konjac.

How it works: Glucomannan absorbs water and becomes gel-like. It "sits" in your gut and promotes a feeling of fullness, helping you eat fewer calories.

Effectiveness: One 2015 clinical trial showed that taking glucomannan for 60 days could lower body weight among participants with overweight, but only if they were consistently taking the supplement.

Other benefits: Glucomannan is a fiber that can feed the friendly bacteria in the intestine. It can also lower fasting blood sugar and blood cholesterol and works effectively against constipation.

Side effects: Glucomannan can cause bloating, flatulence, and soft stools and can interfere with some oral medications if taken at the same time.

It is important to take glucomannan about half an hour before meals, with a glass of water.

8. Meratrim

Meratrim is a relative newcomer on the diet pill market, made from a combination of two plant extracts — Sphaeranthus indicus and Garcinia mangostana — that may change the metabolism of fat cells.

How it works: It claims to make it harder for fat cells to multiply, decrease the amount of fat they pick up from the bloodstream, and help them burn stored fat.

Effectiveness: Very few studies about Meratrim exist. One 2012 study involved 60 people with overweight and placed on a strict 2,000-calorie diet and increased physical activity, with either Meratrim or a placebo. After 16 weeks, the Meratrim group had lost 11 lb (5 kg) and 4 inches (10 centimeters) off their waistlines.

Another study suggested that Meratrim had long-lasting effects on appetite suppression.

Side effects: No side effects have been reported.

9. Green tea extract

Alessio Bogani/Stocksy United

Green tea extract is a popular ingredient in many weight loss supplements. This is because numerous studies have shown that the main antioxidant it contains, EGCG, may aid fat burning.

How it works: Green tea extract is believed to hinder enzymes such as pancreatic lipase, which, when combined with reduced fat absorption, can be an effective way to treat obesity.

Effectiveness: Many human studies have shown that green tea extract, when paired with exercise, can increase fat burning and cause fat loss, especially in the belly area.

Side effects: Green tea extract is generally well tolerated. It does contain some caffeine and may cause symptoms in people who are sensitive to caffeine.

Additionally, all the health benefits of drinking green tea may also apply to green tea extract. Though, keep in mind that while studies showing the benefits of green tea extract use doses of 500 mg per day or more, 1 cup (236 mL) of green tea only contains approximately 50–100 mg of green tea extract.

10. Conjugated linoleic acid (CLA)

CLA has been a popufat-lossloss supplement for years.

It is known as one of the "healthier" trans fats and is found naturally in some fatty animal-derived foods like cheese and butter.

How it works: CLA may reduce appetite, boost metabolism, and stimulate the breakdown of body fat.

Effectiveness: In one study, taking 3,000 mg of CLA per day for 3 months resulted in a significant reduction in body fat mass and body fat percentage, compared to a placebo. However, body weight and BMI were not significantly reduced.

Similarly, an older review from 2012 found CLA was linked with an average weight loss of 1.5 lb (0.7 kg), which the authors note may not be clinically meaningful for people trying to lose weight.

Side effects: CLA can cause various digestive side effects and may have harmful effects over the long term, potentially contributing to fatty liver, insulin resistance, and increased inflammation.

11. Forskolin

Forskolin is an extract from a plant in the mint family that is thought to be effective for weight loss.

How it works: It may raise levels of a compound inside cells called cAMP, which can stimulate fat burning).

Effectiveness: One 2012 study of 30 men with excess weight or obesity showed that forskolin reduced body fat and increased muscle mass while not affecting body weight. Another older study involving 23 women with excess weight found no effects.

More recent, high-quality research on the potential effectiveness of forskolin is needed.

Side effects: There is minimal data on the safety of this supplement or the risk of side effects.

12. Bitter orange/synephrine

A type of orange called bitter orange contains the compound synephrine.

Synephrine is related to ephedrine, which used to be a popular ingredient in various weight loss pill formulations.

However, the FDA has since banned ephedrine as a weight-loss ingredient because of serious side effects.

How it works: Synephrine has similar mechanisms to ephedrine but is less potent. It could help reduce appetite and increase fat burning.

Effectiveness: Very few studies have been done on synephrine, but one older review reported that ephedrine can cause significant short-term weight loss.

On the other hand, a more recent 2022 review of 18 studies concluded that synephrine was not effective for weight loss and may increase blood pressure and heart rate with prolonged use.

Side effects: Like ephedrine, synephrine may have serious side effects related to the heart. It may also have a high risk of dependence.

When to talk with a doctor

If you've tried everything to lose weight and the scale still won't budge, it's worth talking with a healthcare professional, like a doctor or registered dietitian, about whether a weight loss medication might be right for you.

Because these pills can have serious side effects and are not safe for everyone, it's important not to take any weight loss drugs or supplements without consulting a professional first.

Some digital weight loss platforms, including Ro and Calibrate, include GLP-1 medications in their treatment plans for people who meet certain eligibility criteria.

You can read our comprehensive reviews of Calibrate and Ro Health to learn more.

Heads up

Weight loss drugs may not be recommended for people with eating disorders (EDs), even if they are at higher body weights, as there is a risk of misuse of prescription or over-the-counter diet drugs.

Studies also suggest that people with higher body weights are disproportionately likely to experience disordered eating and eating disorder symptoms.

If you are preoccupied with food or weight, feel guilt surrounding your food choices, or routinely engage in restrictive diets, consider reaching out for support. These behaviors may indicate a disordered relationship with food or an ED.

Disordered eating and EDs can affect anyone, regardless of gender identity, race, age, body size, socioeconomic status, or other identities.

They can be caused by any combination of biological, social, cultural, and environmental factors — not just by exposure to diet culture.

Feel empowered to talk with a qualified healthcare professional, such as a registered dietitian, if you're managing any of these behaviors.

You can also chat, call, or text anonymously with trained volunteers at the National Eating Disorders Association helpline for free or explore the organization's free and low-cost resources.

Frequently asked questions

How effective are weight loss drugs?

Weight loss medications and supplements can vary in effectiveness.

Some prescription drugs have been shown to cause significant weight loss. However, research is limited on the effectiveness of many OTC supplements, and some studies have even found that certain products — such as synephrine and forskolin — are unlikely to have a significant impact on body weight.

In addition to which specific weight loss drug you use, individual results can vary based on many other factors, including your diet, health status, and activity level.

Which weight loss medications are best for weight loss?

The best weight loss drug for you depends on your weight loss goals, health status, and personal preferences. Though prescription medications like GLP-1 agonists are supported by stronger research and are more likely to be effective, they may also be associated with adverse side effects and risks.

Keep in mind that regardless of which supplement or medication you choose, it's important to follow a well-rounded diet and healthy lifestyle. In addition to maximizing your potential results, it can increase the likelihood of maintaining weight loss long-term.

Does insurance cover prescription weight loss medications?

If considered medically necessary, insurance companies may cover certain prescription weight loss medications. Some manufacturers also offer savings cards, which can help lower the cost of your co-pay.

The bottom line

Many weight loss medications and supplements are available, including prescription and over-the-counter options. Overall, prescription medications have stronger evidence to support their effectiveness for meaningful weight loss.

A doctor or other trusted healthcare professional can help you determine which is right for you and how to incorporate it into a healthy weight management plan.

However, it's important to remember that these medications and supplements should not be considered a "quick fix" for weight loss.

Instead, they should be used only as directed and paired with a balanced diet, healthy lifestyle, and regular physical activity for best results.

CONCLUSION

it gives you the instruments to be the repairman of your well-being, telling you the best way to tweak your dietary patterns and way of life to shed pounds economically and feel perfect as long as possible.

You don't need to put on weight as you age. That is the basic yet progressive commitment of The Entire Body Reset, which uncovers why standard eating regimens and exercise counsel quit working for us as we approach midlife — and uncovers how straightforward changes to the manner in which we eat can end, and, surprisingly, turn around, age-related weight gain and muscle misfortune.

The Entire Body Reset presents dazzling new proof about the force of "protein timing" for individuals at midlife — research that blows away momentum government rules, disproves the fantasy of easing back digestion systems and "unavoidable" weight gain, and has an impact on the way individuals in their mid-forties and more established ought to contemplate food. The Entire Body Reset makes sense of in basic, motivating terms precisely the way that our bodies change with age, and how eating to oblige those changes can cause us to answer practice as though we were twenty to thirty years more youthful

www.ingramcontent.com/pod-product-compliance
Lightning Source LLC
Chambersburg PA
CBHW070612220526
45467CB00003B/1394